Mental Health Guide

for

Elderly Women

Uncover your mental health management tips
and guide for 2024

Gilbert Predmore

A Book carefully carved by

Gilbert Predmore

Index

Introduction

Being older may be a rewarding and demanding experience, particularly for women who must deal with shifting roles, cultural expectations, and life experience. This handbook provides useful resources and perspectives to assist senior women in managing their emotional health. It offers a secure environment for investigating encounters, materials, and methods to foster inner serenity and happiness in their elderly years. Since later life affords the chance to reclaim one's voice, prioritize needs, and enjoy a meaningful present, age is not a barrier to mental wellbeing.

Any older woman, regardless of origin, views, or experiences, should use this handbook. In addition to offering evidence-based tactics and empathetic counsel to support mental health and live their best lives on their own terms, it honors the complexity and resiliency of their journey.

Although the twilight years are often seen as a time of development and rediscovery, many elderly women find that they are really a time of tremendous growth and rediscovery. The handbook gives readers the skills and assurance they need to handle these difficulties with poise and discernment.

Author's Preface

I discovered Nana Rachel in her rose garden, a sun-dappled oasis. Her eyes were surrounded by lines made by laughing, each one bearing witness to a life well lived. She was a bright splash of fuchsia at eighty-seven, flourishing against a background of cultural expectations that tend to fade with age.

Adversity was nothing new to Nana Rachel. She had endured physical illnesses, loneliness, and bereavement. Her laughter, however, echoed like wind chimes on a little breeze, her spirit unbowed. She spoke about "mental cobwebs" that attempted to cling, about days clouded by uncertainty, but she also talked about the instruments she used to drive them out.

She would pat her temple and remark, "Mind, dear, needs tending just like these roses." Remove the negativity, let hope's sunlight enter, and see as it begins to flourish once again."

She blossomed, too. With her laughing driving ducks into the reeds, Nana Rachel spent her days taking walks along the river. At the senior center, where she studied tango, the shimmer of the disco light caught her sequined dress like a thousand trapped rainbows. She even started writing poetry online, creating resilient and joyful tapestries with her words.

My inspiration was Nana Rachel. Her narrative serves as a tribute to the unwavering spirit that, at whatever age, everyone of us has. You'll find echoes of her wisdom, useful tools to support your mental health, and gentle proddings to locate your inner vivid music in this book.

In order to experience mental blossom, flip the page, my dear reader, and let Nana Rachel—the dancing queen of the rose garden—to lead the way. Never forget that you may always add the colors of pleasure, resiliency, and hope to your own sunset.

Chapter 1

Overview Of Elderly Women's Mental Health

Common Mental Health Issues Of Elderly Women

Depression

An important mental health problem, depression affects up to 20% of older women worldwide. It is characterized by a chronic melancholy and disinterest, which may take many different forms, including a sense of emptiness or numbness, a loss of enjoyment, and a dismal, despairing sensation. This primary symptom sets depression apart from typical sorrow or loss, which are transitory emotions often triggered by particular experiences. Comprehending this pivotal attribute is imperative in identifying and tackling sadness in elderly ladies, enabling them and their companions to pursue suitable assistance and therapy to recapture the happiness and significance that despair may rob. Depression may be a quiet but powerful ally, particularly for older women. The main features of depression in later life are outlined in this book, along with its many expressions, possible causes, and significant effects on mental health.

Major myths about depression include the following: it's simply sadness, it's a sign of weakness, it's easily controlled with willpower, talking about depression makes it worse, and it's just about feeling sad. In order to properly manage depression, elderly women should prioritize self-care, seek out professional assistance, investigate treatment alternatives, think about taking medication, create a support system, and engage in self-compassion exercises.

For depression to be properly managed, early diagnosis and therapy are critical. A mental health expert should be consulted for an appropriate diagnosis and a customized treatment plan. Positive coping mechanisms and negative thinking patterns may be addressed with the use of several therapeutic modalities, including cognitive-behavioral therapy (CBT) and interpersonal therapy (IPT). Antidepressant drugs may help control brain chemistry and lessen the symptoms of depression, but it's crucial to speak with a doctor to find the right drug and dose for you.

Ultimately, reclaiming control over your life and finding pleasure again requires engaging in self-compassion practices and realizing that recovery is a journey rather than a destination. Don't be afraid to ask for assistance; depression is curable and reversible with the correct services and support.

Depression can appear differently in older adults compared to younger people. Here are some key traits of sadness in the later stages of life:

1. Atypical presentation:

Emphasis on physical symptoms: Older elderly women with depression may come with more physical complaints like aches and pains, tiredness, stomach issues, and sleep problems, rather than the standard emotional symptoms like sadness and loss of interest. This can make it harder to identify sadness, as these signs can also be caused by other physical problems.

Cognitive changes: Depression can be linked with cognitive loss and memory problems in older people. This can lead to a misunderstanding of dementia or Alzheimer's disease.

2. Loss and grief:

Loss of loved ones: Experiencing grief, especially the loss of a spouse or close friend, is a big risk factor for sadness in older people.

Loss of freedom: Facing physical limits or chronic health problems can lead to a loss of independence and a sense of hopelessness, adding to sadness.

Retirement: Retirement can be a major life change that can lead to feelings of isolation and loss of purpose, causing sadness.

3. Social isolation:

Loneliness and social isolation: Older elderly women who live alone or have limited social contact are more likely to experience sadness. This can be due to things like physical limits, transportation problems, or hearing loss.

Negative social interactions: Ageism and discrimination can also add to sadness in older people.

4. Increased risk factors:

Chronic health conditions: Having chronic health conditions like heart disease, diabetes, or cancer can increase the risk of sadness.

Drugs: Certain drugs, such as painkillers and stimulants, can have side effects that add to depression.

Substance abuse: Older elderly women are more likely to misuse alcohol or prescription drugs to cope with depression, which can worsen symptoms in the long run.

It's important to know that sadness is manageable at any age. If you are worried about yourself or an older loved one, please reach out to a mental health professional for help. Early identification and treatment can make a major difference in better quality of life.

A Memoir of Depression:Maria's Narrative

Once a brilliant artist, Maria was well-known for her sun-drenched landscape paintings, but she had lost her identity. The corner easel remained in place, its canvas gathering dust. The laughter that had once filled her little workshop has given way to an enduring quiet, broken only by the hollow echo of her own hopelessness.

Maria's world had lost its color as depression had entered her life like a robber in the night. The excitement of catching a moment of light, or the delight of blending colors, felt like far-off recollections. The brush was heavy in her palm now, every stroke serving as a reminder of the ecstasy she was no longer able to experience.

Her days blended together like a grayscale tapestry. Once a welcoming haven, sleep turned into a prison for her as her own thoughts and dreams tormented her evenings. The world beyond her window seems subdued, with the streets she had known for so long without any charm.

Loved ones' faces seemed far away, and an unseen wall muffled their words. Once a source of joy, social events became intolerable, her anguish being too fresh for the forced grins and upbeat conversation.

However, there was still a glimmer of hope inside in Maria's spirit. It was a little flame that was almost perceptible in the shadows, yet it would not go out. It was the recollection of the person she used to be—the creative who saw beauty in every stroke of paint and the companion who made her sides hurt with laughter.

Despite its fragility, the flicker ended up serving as her beacon. Maria went for assistance, strengthened by the love and support of those close to her. It was not an easy road. On other days, it seemed like the road to recovery would never end and the darkness would swallow her whole.

But the colors gradually, hardly perceptibly, started to reappear. Her paintings gradually began to reclaim the brightness they had lost with a hesitant brushstroke here and a bright yellow splash there. Though tentative at first, the laughter began to seep through her suffering.

Maria's tale serves as a tribute to the human spirit's tenacity and a lesson that optimism may blossom even in the most dire circumstances. Long-lasting shadows may be cast by depression, but it need not define us. One brushstroke at a time, we can restore the colors of our life if we have the guts, the support system, and the appropriate resources.

Anxiety Disorder

A class of mental diseases known as anxiety disorders is defined by excessive concern, anxiousness, and dread. These emotions may seem to have no apparent reason, or they may be brought on by certain circumstances or items. Anxiety may have a substantial negative influence on a person's quality of life and present itself in a variety of physical and mental manifestations.

Anxiety disorders are characterized by excessive concern and dread, which may be brought on by commonplace events like relationships, economics, or the workplace. Anxious elderly women may also have severe phobias of certain things or circumstances, such spiders, heights, or public speaking. Anxiety may manifest physically as an elevated heart rate, fast breathing, perspiration, tense muscles, headaches, upset stomach, lightheadedness, and exhaustion.

Anxiety-related behavioral changes, such as avoidance, safety seeking, and compulsions, might happen. When anxiety gets out of control, it may make it hard for a person to go about their everyday life, work, go to school, maintain relationships, and enjoy hobbies.

Sarah, a graphic artist who battles generalized anxiety disorder (GAD), is a real-life example of someone dealing with an anxiety condition. When she is under pressure to complete a significant client presentation by a certain date, her worry turns into panic attacks. Sarah employs the relaxation methods she acquired in therapy to control her anxiety. These techniques include deep breathing, positive affirmations, and visualizing a serene and tranquil area.

Myths about anxiety disorders might prevent elderly women from getting the support they need to properly manage their symptoms. Commonly held beliefs about anxiety include the following: it's all in your brain, it's simply a mental illness, medicine is the only way to treat it, cognitive-behavioral therapy (CBT) is the only way to treat it, and those who suffer from anxiety are weak or unable.

In order to properly manage anxiety, elderly women should see a professional, look into treatment choices, think about taking medication when required, take care of themselves, learn relaxation methods, create a support system, and stand up for themselves. elderly women may overcome the difficulties brought on by anxiety disorders and learn to lead full lives by realizing the value of getting assistance and controlling their symptoms.

In summary, anxiety disorders are a difficult and crippling mental condition that may be managed with the correct help and knowledge. elderly women may better manage their symptoms and lead satisfying lives by getting professional assistance, looking into treatment choices, thinking about taking medication, practicing self-care, learning relaxation methods, creating a support system, and standing up for themselves.

Dementia

Memory, reasoning, problem-solving, language, visual perception, and executive function are just a few of the cognitive domains that are affected by dementia, a gradual loss in cognitive function that has a substantial influence on day-to-day functioning. It is a phrase used to describe a collection of symptoms brought on by a number of different underlying brain illnesses, such as frontotemporal dementia, vascular dementia, Lewy body dementia, and Alzheimer's disease.

There are techniques to control dementia symptoms and enhance quality of life; it is not a typical aspect of aging. Dementia patients should be treated with respect and compassion since they are still unique persons with distinct experiences and viewpoints. Speak with a healthcare provider if you or someone you know is worried about dementia for a diagnosis and advice on what services and support alternatives are available.

Individuals and families may manage the path of dementia with bravery and dignity if they get an early diagnosis, the right support, and understanding. Dementia is a journey, not a destination. The idea that dementia is just forgetfulness and a natural aspect of aging, the idea that dementia sufferers are burdens and ought to be institutionalized, the idea that there is no hope for dementia sufferers, and the idea that dementia sufferers are incapable of communicating are common misconceptions regarding dementia.

Although successful medications and treatments may control symptoms, reduce the course of dementia, and enhance quality of life, dementia is ultimately an incurable disorder. Medication, cognitive-behavioral treatment, and non-pharmacological methods such as music therapy and recollection therapy are among examples.

Maintaining relationships and fostering connections may be facilitated by learning good communication techniques, exercising tolerance and understanding, and concentrating on emotions and shared experiences while communicating with someone who has dementia.

Making financial and legal plans for the future may help elderly women with dementia and their family make choices and make sure their desires are honored. A seamless transition to future requirements may be ensured and peace of mind can be gained by openly addressing future care choices, establishing legal documentation, and including loved ones in the planning process.

Together, let's make dementia a reality that is compassionately accepted, understood, and supported.

PTSD

The symptoms of post-traumatic stress disorder (PTSD) include severe and intrusive reliving of a traumatic experience, along with symptoms that greatly affect day-to-day functioning. These recollections might show up as a variety of symptoms, including as nightmares, intrusive thoughts, emotional triggers, hypervigilance, avoidance, depressive shifts in mood and cognitive patterns, and shifts in emotional and physical reactions.

Not only war or battle, but any kind of stressful incident may result in PTSD. Numerous events, such as natural catastrophes, accidents, physical or sexual assault, and simply witnessing abuse or violence, might contribute to it. Improving quality of life and controlling PTSD symptoms need early diagnosis and therapy. Therapy, such as cognitive-behavioral therapy (CBT), and medication, when necessary, are effective forms of treatment.

Misconceptions about Post-Traumatic Stress Disorder (PTSD) often prevent elderly women from getting the treatment they need and make recovery more difficult. It is crucial to dispel common misconceptions and investigate ways to increase knowledge and effective assistance in order to create understanding.

Myth 1: Only first responders and veterans of combat suffer from PTSD.
Reality: Anybody who has gone through a traumatic incident, such as an accident, a natural catastrophe, abuse, or violence, might get PTSD. fostering open dialogue about trauma and its repercussions in order to reduce stigma and raise awareness that PTSD is a condition that affects elderly women of all backgrounds.

Myth2: Individuals suffering from PTSD are feigned or weak.
Reality: PTSD is not a sign of weakness; rather, it is a complicated mental health disease. Disprove victim-blaming stories and highlight PTSD's scientific foundation. Promote compassion and understanding for those who are managing a difficult illness.

Myth number three: "Just get over it" and "Time will heal all wounds."
Reality: Individualized, evidence-based therapies, such as medication and therapy, are necessary to treat PTSD; it does not go away on its own. Encourage the use of mental health services and raise awareness of the benefits of expert PTSD treatments.

Myth 4: Discussing the experience will exacerbate it.
Reality: Talking about the incident with others in a secure and encouraging setting may be healing and aid in the trauma's processing. Pacing and individual limits, however, must be respected.

Myth 5: Medicine is a temporary cure and is addicting.
Reality: In addition to treatment, medication may be a useful aid for controlling PTSD symptoms. Dispel the myths surrounding medicine by providing factual details on its ability to treat PTSD symptoms and promote general healing.

For those suffering from PTSD, creating a supportive atmosphere is essential. Promoting healthy coping strategies like exercise and relaxation techniques, fighting isolation, pushing for workplace support and accommodations for elderly women with disabilities, and opposing discriminatory attitudes and policies can all contribute to the development of a society in which elderly women with PTSD feel empowered to ask for assistance, obtain the resources they need, and set out on the road to healing and recovery.

Protective & Resilient Factors

As we get older, life offers new chances and difficulties, which emphasizes the need of maintaining mental health. This manual examines resilient and protective elements that might aid older women's journeys toward mental wellness.

Core Protective Factors:
Develop ties with your loved ones, friends, and neighborhood associations. In addition to preventing loneliness and offering emotional support, social interaction promotes a feeling of purpose and belonging. Social dynamics may shift as elderly women age, making it more crucial than ever to preserve deep connections.

Elderly women often have particular difficulties, such as physical impairments, widowhood, or living alone, which may result in loneliness and social isolation. Robust social networks operate as a buffer against these difficulties. A feeling of satisfaction, purpose, and belonging may be facilitated by engaging in community events, keeping strong connections, and partaking in social activities. These relationships provide chances for emotional support, friendship, and shared experiences. Frequent **Social connection**[1] may also improve mood, lower stress levels, and enhance cognitive performance.

Strong social ties become apparent as a bright thread woven throughout the wellbeing of older women as life progresses. They provide a strong defense against life's obstacles as well as a lively source of happiness and meaning.

Defying loneliness and isolation: Growing older may exacerbate feelings of loneliness, steal happiness, and accelerate mental deterioration. Good social ties serve as a warm hug that chases away loneliness and gives one a feeling of community and belonging. Laughter over a cup of tea or heated debates in a book club are examples of regular encounters with loved ones that provide a safe haven against the cold of solitude.

Enhancing cognitive function and halting cognitive aging: Social engagement serves as a mental exercise, keeping the mind active and focused. Engaging in lively discussions, debating current events, or playing cooperative card games enhances cognitive functions and lowers the likelihood of dementia and cognitive decline.

It takes time and work to build solid relationships, but it is imperative that older women embrace technology, make new friends, contribute their time and skills, and reconnect with old ones.

Having supportive social networks that provide security, happiness, and a feeling of community is not a luxury but rather a need. To improve your life and the lives of elderly women around you, reach out, connect, and enjoy the brilliant colors of social contact.

Taking part in worthwhile pursuits like volunteering, taking up a new hobby, or picking up new skills may provide one a feeling of satisfaction, pleasure, and purpose that can improve one's general well-being. These are worthwhile pursuits that enhance one's well being on a personal level. For older women, taking part in meaningful activities has a multitude of positive effects on their wellbeing, making it a potent protective factor.

In later stages of life, **Meaningful activities[2]** help build a rewarding lifestyle, preserve physical well-being, enhance identity and self-esteem, increase mood and cognitive function, and fight loneliness and isolation. Creative endeavors, physical exercise, social interaction, lifelong learning, and spiritual practices are a few examples of meaningful activities.

For older women, **Physical health**[3] is an additional essential aspect that encompasses a range of factors that contribute to overall well-being. It entails leading a healthy lifestyle by engaging in routine exercise, eating a balanced diet, and getting enough sleep. Sufficient physical well-being cultivates resilience, suppleness, and strength, allowing women to effortlessly handle everyday tasks. A healthy body strengthens the immune system, extends life, and helps avoid age-related illnesses. Elderly women who prioritize their physical health may have more energy, a lower chance of developing chronic diseases, and a better capacity to have active, meaningful lives as they age.

Maintaining physical health goes beyond just being mobile and active; it is a strong defense against many obstacles and lays the foundation for a happy, satisfying life. Following are a few advantages of maintaining your physical health:

1. Increasing Resilience: Consistent exercise lowers the risk of falls, enhances balance and coordination, and fortifies muscles and bones. This translates into increased resilience and independence, giving you the confidence to handle everyday chores.

2. Improving Well-Being: Engaging in physical exercise releases endorphins, which are the body's natural feel-good chemicals that help you feel happier and more hopeful by reducing stress and anxiety. This optimistic mindset enhances general well-being by influencing other facets of life.

3. Empowering Independence: Maintaining your physical health enables you to be independent and active, carrying out everyday duties without assistance from others. This feeling of independence and control over your life gives you self-worth and confidence, enabling you to live life as you see fit.

4. Promoting Social Connection: Participating in group activities gives you the chance to meet elderly women and form connections with like-minded people. By fostering a feeling of connection and belonging, this social engagement fights loneliness and isolation.

Confidence building: Engaging in physical activities may help you feel more confident and good about yourself, which will make you feel more at ease interacting with others and doing new things.

Recall that putting your physical health first is a lifetime process rather than a final goal. Build a schedule that suits you step by step by starting small and engaging in things you like. Your body, mind, and soul are strengthened with each step you take toward physical well-being, giving you the ability to live a long, healthy, and meaningful life.

For older women, having a **Good self-image**[4] is crucial because it encourages perseverance and an appreciation for their distinct life experiences. It encourages development and change by opposing the conventional propensity to see aging as a decline. It fosters self-compassion, enabling elderly women to accept flaws, provide forgiveness, and rejoice in victories. This promotes self-worth and inner tranquility.

A good view of oneself encourages healthy decision-making, draws favorable events, and increases confidence. It encourages elderly women to give priority to pursuits that enhance their bodily and mental well-being. Positive self-images, however, are cyclical and not static. Elderly women may grow a strong inner garden with the fortitude to overcome obstacles and the insight to enjoy life's journey by tending to these seedlings.

Another important quality for senior women is **Optimism**[5], which enables them to face life's challenges head-on with power and elegance. It is a mental strength that enables women to approach challenges with optimism. When presented with challenges, optimists are more likely to use constructive coping mechanisms, which lower stress and enhance mental wellness. Additionally, they are more resilient, which serves as a protective barrier against stress and negativity and enables them to overcome failures with optimism.

Optimism promotes healthy behaviors like exercise and a balanced diet, which are connected to improved physical health outcomes. Optimistic elderly women also tend to have stronger social networks because their upbeat attitude and openness to social interaction draw others and create stronger bonds, which are essential for emotional support and a feeling of community.

In conclusion, for older women to overcome obstacles in life and discover meaning and purpose in their lives, optimism and a good self-image are essential.

Among the most powerful and durable forces in the lives of senior women is **Gratitude**[6]. It promotes changing one's viewpoint so that one may concentrate on life's positive aspects and little pleasures despite its difficulties. This gratitude fosters optimism, nurtures well-being, and acts as a barrier against negativity.

Gratitude helps us get over the inevitable aches and pains of aging, the losses that come with time, and future worries by encouraging us to concentrate on the positive, the little pleasures, and the bright spots. The sun's warmth on our skin, the joy of our grandkids, and the knowledge accumulated through years of experience all call us to relish them. This change of viewpoint encourages satisfaction and inner serenity even in the midst of hardship.
Choosing to be grateful means actively identifying and enjoying all of life's blessings, no matter how little. When we repeat something again and over, it develops our optimism muscle, which enables us to see the bright side of things, even in trying circumstances, and to have faith that things will eventually get better. This upbeat perspective strengthens our fortitude and helps us go on in the face of difficulties.

Gratitude boosts our immune system, reduces stress hormones, and enhances the quality of our sleep, among other positive effects on our wellbeing. It reminds us that we are not alone and that our lives have significance, which gives us a feeling of direction and meaning. This improved well-being serves as the cornerstone of our resilience, enabling us to face challenges head-on and deal with the intricacies of aging with courage and grace.

Gratitude is ingrained in daily life and doesn't need elaborate displays of appreciation. Keeping a gratitude diary, spreading appreciation, appreciating the little things in life, and engaging in mindfulness exercises are a few ways older women may integrate it into their daily routines.

Practicing gratitude makes it a natural reaction that helps us weather life's ups and downs. Gratitude is a journey, not a destination.

Promoting Support For Elderly Women Mental Health

The mental health of elderly women is particularly vulnerable to issues stemming from ageism, social isolation, and cultural expectations. These problems may make mental health conditions like anxiety and despair worse, warping their sense of purpose and pleasure. A comprehensive strategy that places a high value on community and connection is required to overcome these issues. Promoting social engagement, fostering current relationships, giving volunteer opportunities, using technology to combat loneliness, helping with transportation, and pairing volunteers with senior ladies for company and discussion are some solutions. Creating a network of social workers, healthcare providers, and community volunteers can provide comprehensive assistance. Elderly women might be encouraged to seek treatment without feeling ashamed by encouraging candid talks about mental health within the community.

The socioeconomic determinants of mental health, such as financial stability, access to cheap housing, and quality healthcare, may also be addressed via advocacy and legislative reforms. We can enable older women to travel the road of mental well-being, surrounded by the warmth of connection and the strength of community, by tackling these issues and putting innovative solutions into practice.

Two major obstacles that prevent older women from getting the mental health care they need are **ageism** and **stigma.** Certain preconceived notions about older women, such as their fragility, incapacity, or lack of mental ability, might contribute to the idea that mental health issues are "normal" or "inevitable." Discrimination in healthcare settings may also be a major obstacle, with issues being taken seriously enough or being written off as age-related.

On the flip side, stigma is the deeply held conviction that mental illness is a weakness, which causes guilt, fear of being judged, and a reluctance to talk to others about mental health issues. Myths about "normal aging" might deter elderly women from getting the care they need and from using available resources. Social isolation may make pre-existing mental health issues worse.

Knowledge and awareness campaigns are essential to removing these obstacles. It is critical to increase knowledge regarding the frequency and consequences of mental health problems among older women. Elderly women who share their experiences of resiliency, healing, and wellbeing may dispel harmful preconceptions and encourage others to get the care they need. It is crucial to guarantee that mental health treatments are easily available, reasonably priced, and considerate of the unique requirements of older women.

It may change lives to provide safe locations where senior women can interact, talk about their experiences, and get support from their peers. Individuals may be empowered by support groups to speak out for their own needs and fight stigma in their communities.

For older women, **financial fragility** is an additional difficulty. Many are severely financially vulnerable, which may make it more difficult for them to get treatment and be healthy. The female wage gap, rising healthcare expenditures, caregiving obligations, social isolation, restricted access to resources, and loss of autonomy and dignity are some of the difficulties.

Proposing wage parity and gender equality, increasing access to reasonably priced healthcare, providing assistance to family caregivers, encouraging financial planning and literacy, and fortifying social support systems are a few possible remedies. We can make it easier for older women to prioritize their mental health and well-being by

recognizing the difficulties they experience, fighting for institutional improvements, and encouraging support from friends and family.
Creating a network of support is crucial for alleviating loneliness and promoting relationships for the mental health of older women.

For older women, **loneliness** is a serious problem that may result in emotions of dejection, worry, and loneliness. A few of the factors that lead to loneliness include stigma, gaps in technology, and societal changes. Community involvement, intergenerational initiatives, digital education, mental health awareness, and strengthening personal relationships may all be used to fight loneliness.
Intergenerational programs facilitate connection between older women and younger people, while community involvement promotes participation in local events, senior centers, and activity groups. With the aid of technological training, older women may securely and successfully access and use technology, facilitating online connections with friends, family, and communities. Open dialogue about loneliness and mental health is encouraged by mental health awareness, which also empowers older women to access services and seek assistance without feeling judged.

Buddy programs help older women feel less alone by matching them with volunteers or younger elderly women for frequent phone conversations, in-person visits, or activities. Creative expression helps senior women to express themselves via writing, painting, music, or other creative avenues, and pet therapy may lessen feelings of loneliness and despair. Support groups lessen feelings of loneliness by fostering a sense of understanding and connection.

Financial accessibility is essential for supporting the mental health of older women. Among the difficulties include stigmatization, little awareness, and restricted finances. Increasing the availability of public healthcare, expanding the scope of reasonably priced community-based services, using technology, increasing awareness, and enabling financial stability are some of the solutions. Peer support groups, intergenerational initiatives, and innovative fundraisers are examples of inventive solutions.

Elderly women may have fulfilling lives with meaningful relationships if we address the underlying causes of loneliness, empower people, and build connections.

Encouraging older women to get mental health care requires financial accessibility. A multimodal strategy including healthcare access, cost, awareness, and social support is required to solve this problem. Peer support groups may be a useful tool for creating a secure environment where elderly women can share their experiences, provide support to one another, and feel less alone.

Peer support groups provide a secure space where women may freely talk about their experiences, dispelling stigma and giving them the confidence to ask for assistance. Through tools, anecdotes, and shared coping mechanisms, they also foster empowerment and resilience. Group activities that emphasize mindfulness practices, relaxation methods, or healthy behaviors might motivate women to put their physical and mental health first.

Socialization is an additional advantage of peer support groups. They provide chances for social contact, help fight isolation and loneliness, and share information and advocacy campaigns. Peer support groups that work well should have inclusive, varied memberships and be led by skilled facilitators. It is important to create respect and confidentiality and to provide access to resources.

While peer support groups may be a beneficial addition to individual treatment, they should not be used in lieu of professional mental health care. Peer support groups provide safe venues for interaction, experience sharing, and mutual support, and they may be an important part of older women's mental health care. We can create a world where every old woman may have a full life by ending the stigma, creating supportive networks, and making sure she gets the care she needs.

Early Warning Signs of Issues with Mental health

Early detection of mental health problems is essential for getting treatment in a timely manner and avoiding consequences. Changes in mood and emotions, such as depression or anxiety, as well as chronic melancholy, despair, or anger, are common warning signs to be aware of. Tearfulness, lack of motivation, or an overall sense of emptiness are some manifestations of these symptoms.

Another serious warning sign is hopelessness, which may encourage further seclusion and withdrawal and make it more difficult to ask for assistance. Another indicator of underlying stress, anxiety, or depression is irritability, which may exacerbate relationship problems and make day-to-day living more challenging. Since these symptoms might occur in combination, it is important to determine their degree and duration.

Keep an eye out for behavioral shifts, such as retreating from social interactions, skipping out on obligations, or losing interest in past interests. Unusual outbursts or adjustments in how you control your anger might be signs of deeper problems.

It's critical to treat excessive anger or hostility carefully since it may indicate a number of mental health problems. Anger out of control may cause friction and harm to relationships in both the personal and professional spheres. Outbursts may also cause mental and physical injury, which can result in property destruction, self-harm, or aggressive behavior against others. Anger management issues, such as borderline personality disorder, depression, anxiety, PTSD, and intermittent explosive disorder (IED), may also be contributing factors to excessive anger.

Seeking professional assistance from a therapist or counselor is crucial when you see excessive anger. You should also use self-regulation methods like mindfulness, relaxation exercises, and anger management techniques. Developing strong support networks and taking care of the underlying issue are two important strategies for anger management.

Apathy toward employment, interests, or social connections may be a serious indicator of mental health problems. Losing interest in things you used to enjoy may cause feelings of emptiness, loneliness, and a lack of drive, all of which are detrimental to well being. Numerous mental health disorders, such as depression, anxiety, burnout, and trauma, have been linked to this symptom.

Examine the length and intensity of the changes, together with any accompanying symptoms and underlying reasons, to determine if a persistent loss of interest is indicative of a possible mental health problem. An expert in mental health may assess the circumstances, pinpoint any underlying problems, and suggest suitable courses of action.
Recall that losing interest in things you used to like might be a sign of a curable mental health illness rather than a weakness or defect in your character. For the purpose of treating mental health issues and enhancing general wellbeing, early intervention is essential. Asking for assistance is a brave and strong move.

Severe mood swings, especially those that occur quickly, may be a serious indicator of a number of mental health problems. These mood fluctuations may take many different forms, including intense anxiety and serenity, irritation and withdrawal, and melancholy and mania. The regularity and severity of these mood swings matter because they have a big effect on day-to-day activities, interpersonal interactions, and the workplace.

It is essential to seek professional assistance, engage in self-care, establish a support network, and keep in mind that you are not alone in order to handle these symptoms. Mental health problems are widespread, and getting treatment may significantly impact both managing mental health problems and enhancing general wellbeing.

A shift in thought or behavior may also be a sign of mental health problems. Ignoring social commitments or avoiding friends and relatives might be indicators of anxiety or depression. Isolation or social disengagement from activities may be serious warning signs of mental problems that make social interaction seem burdensome or unfeasible. Anxiety, sadness, and other mental health issues may be made worse by isolation, which can result in loneliness.

Abrupt or dramatic shifts in social disengagement are important because they may point to a more severe problem. In order to resolve this, show them your care and compassion, urge them to ask for assistance, provide helpful advice, and put them in touch with available resources.

Indications of stress, anxiety, or depression include trouble falling asleep, frequent awakenings, and excessive tiredness. Our physical and mental health depend heavily on our sleep habits, so when those patterns drastically alter, it may be an indication of underlying mental health problems. While occasional sleep problems are common, persistent or notable changes should be taken carefully and evaluated with a medical provider.

Establish a regular sleep schedule, develop a calming bedtime ritual, abstain from caffeine and alcohol before bed, make sure your bedroom is cool, dark, and quiet, get regular exercise—just avoid intense activity right before bed—and, if you're still having trouble falling asleep after 20 minutes, engage in soothing activities until you feel tired. Speak with your physician or a mental health specialist if you have concerns about your sleep habits. They can assist in determining the root cause of your issues and an efficient course of action.

To sum up, controlling mental health concerns and enhancing general wellbeing may be facilitated by identifying and treating behavioral changes, mood swings, and sleep patterns. In order to maintain a healthy and balanced lifestyle, it is imperative that anyone suffering these symptoms get expert assistance and support.

Focus issues may be an early indicator of a number of mental health issues, including ADHD, depression, and anxiety. It is critical to take into account the intensity and length of the attention issues, in addition to any other symptoms including behavioral abnormalities, mood swings, sleep issues, or changes in appetite. It's also critical to take into account any underlying medical or mental health issues that can be contributing to the focus issues.

It's critical to get expert assistance to determine the problem and develop workable remedies if your inability to concentrate is chronic and negatively affecting your life. Seek help from loved ones and experts, and be kind and patient with yourself.

Not merely mental health problems may cause difficulty concentrating; other circumstances can also often cause this symptom. It is crucial to get expert assistance in order to determine the source and develop workable treatments if it is severe, ongoing, and accompanied by additional symptoms. If you are worried about your mental health, don't be afraid to ask for help.

Suicidal or self-harming thoughts or plans should be taken seriously and need to be addressed right away. Take urgent action by talking to someone you trust, getting professional assistance, making a safety plan, and maintaining contact if you or someone you know feels these ideas. Recognize that you are not alone and respect their limits. elderly women exist who are concerned about you and want to support you.

Additionally effective markers of underlying mental health problems are physical changes. Acknowledging these shifts might be essential to getting support and enhancing general wellbeing. Important bodily changes to be aware of include altered energy levels, difficulty sleeping, changes in food and weight, unexplained aches and pains, changes in sexual and digestive functions, changes in skin, hair, and nails, and compromised immune system alterations.

Just because one or two of these are present doesn't always indicate a mental health problem; they are just some broad symptoms. But a combination of these adjustments or notable deviations from your typical state of physical health ought to make you seek medical attention. Finding the root cause of these changes and creating effective treatment strategies might be facilitated by speaking with a physician or mental health specialist. Ignoring physical warning indicators might exacerbate symptoms of mental illness and result in consequences.

Maintaining your physical health is crucial to your mental wellness. You may have a happier and more balanced life by learning to listen to your body's cues and getting assistance when you need it.

Chapter 2

Techniques for preserving Mental health of Elderly Women

Developing resilience and coping skills

Chapter One delves into protective and resilient factors that improve the mental health of elderly women. Key factors to consider include internal factors such as social connections, positive self-image, coping skills, physical health, age-friendly environments, access to healthcare, financial security, and combating ageism and discrimination.

Internal factors include strong social networks, which provide emotional support and a sense of belonging. Positive self-image can be achieved through reminiscing about past accomplishments, learning new skills, and engaging in activities that bring joy and purpose. Coping skills involve equipping women with healthy coping mechanisms like relaxation techniques, mindfulness exercises, or journaling to manage stress and negative emotions effectively. Physical health can be significantly impacted by regular exercise, balanced diet, and adequate sleep. Age-friendly environments create safe and accessible spaces that cater to the specific needs of elderly women, promoting independence and reducing falls risk.

Access to healthcare is crucial for addressing potential issues early on, and financial stability can reduce stress and anxiety. Proactive financial planning and access to necessary resources are also essential. Challenges to ageism and discrimination can contribute to a more inclusive and respectful environment that contributes to mental well-being.

As life's tapestry unfolds, elderly women face unique challenges that can test their mental fortitude. Yet, within them lies an innate resilience waiting to be nurtured and strengthened. Techniques for coping skills to safeguard their mental well-being include developing healthy coping mechanisms through creative outlets like painting, writing, or music. Visual impressions can help ignite interest in building healthy coping mechanisms for elderly women.

Metaphors and stories can be used to illustrate these coping mechanisms. For example, weaving a tapestry can symbolize healing through self-care practices like positive affirmations, mindfulness exercises, and connecting with loved ones. Sharing a story of a seasoned captain navigating through rough seas can represent the importance of resourcefulness and resilience in navigating life's challenges. The Blooming Desert can symbolize the strength and resourcefulness of elderly women even in challenging circumstances.

Interactive activities can include a coping mechanism collage, a "Strength Story" Sharing Circle, and mindful movement workshops. By sparking curiosity, empowering agency, and creating a sense of possibility, these strategies can make healthy coping mechanisms engaging, relevant, and ultimately effective for elderly women on their journey towards mental well-being.

Regular exercise is a powerful tool for both mental and physical well-being, as it releases endorphins, improves mood, and combats cognitive decline. Exercise can be a transformative force for mental and emotional well-being, as it releases endorphins, which naturally combat stress and anxiety. It can also help boost mood by releasing endorphins, which are feel-good chemicals that naturally combat stress and anxiety.

Physical activity can also be a mood booster, helping to combat loneliness and isolation. The rhythmic movements and increased blood flow can elevate mood, leaving you feeling more energetic and optimistic. It's a natural way to combat loneliness and isolation, especially if you join a group fitness class or find an exercise buddy.

Confidence building is another benefit of regular physical activity. As you build strength and flexibility, you'll accomplish things you might not have thought possible, fostering a sense of pride and accomplishment. This newfound confidence can spill over into other areas of your life, helping you tackle challenges with a more positive attitude.

Sleep enhancement is another benefit of physical activity. Exercise helps regulate your sleep cycle, making it easier to fall asleep and stay asleep throughout the night. Social interaction is vital for mental health, and having a supportive network can provide encouragement and make exercise more enjoyable.

To incorporate physical activity into your daily routine, find an activity you enjoy, start slow and gradually increase the intensity and duration of your workouts. Set realistic goals and celebrate your achievements, no matter how small. Find a workout buddy or join a fitness class for extra motivation and support.

By making physical activity a regular part of your life, you're investing in your physical and mental well-being.

Developing skills to address challenges constructively and plan for the future can empower elderly women to navigate difficulties with confidence. Practicing problem-solving techniques can bolster resilience.

Developing healthy coping mechanisms is crucial for everyone, especially for elderly women who might face unique challenges related to aging. Building problem-solving and planning skills can become powerful tools in their mental health toolbox.

Focus on strengths: Acknowledge existing problem-solving abilities, identify existing planning skills, develop new skills, introduce simple problem-solving frameworks, practice planning through role-playing, and use technology as an aid. Promote confidence and independence by celebrating small successes, encouraging taking initiative, and normalizing making mistakes as part of the learning process.

Community and support: Foster peer support groups, connect with family and friends, and access professional resources when needed. Respect individual preferences: Each woman will have her own preferred style of problem-solving and planning. Focus on empowerment: Equip women with skills and confidence to handle life's challenges independently, while also knowing they have access to support if needed.

Celebrate resilience: Highlight the incredible strength and adaptability of elderly women. By empowering them with these tools and fostering an environment of support and understanding, they can navigate life's challenges with confidence and grace, blossoming into a vibrant source of mental well-being.

Developing a Good Behavior

Encouraging senior women's mental health is essential to fostering an atmosphere that is kind and encouraging. It is important to embrace a few crucial actions in order to promote this:

1. Empathy and Respect: Be aware of the particular difficulties someone could be facing as a result of their age, health, or experiences. Be kind and empathetic to all women, but particularly to older women who may have particular difficulties.

2. Actively Listen: Make eye contact, keep your posture open, and focus entirely on the task at hand without interruptions. Reaffirm their emotions by saying something like, "That sounds difficult," or "I can understand why you might feel that way." Avoid interjecting or giving uninvited advice unless you are specifically requested.

3. Speak with empathy: Steer clear of dismissive or judgmental words. Instead, say something like "Tell me more" or "Can you share how you're feeling about that." Sayings like "It seems like you're feeling frustrated" or "That situation must have been very stressful for you" might help you relate to them emotionally.

4. Be Patient and Nonjudgmental: Take into account the possibility that older women may communicate differently or digest information more slowly. Don't push them to answer right away or hurry them. Consider them as distinct elderly women with distinctive viewpoints and experiences. Even if you disagree, show tolerance for differing opinions and respect for their freedom to make their own decisions.

5. Provide helpful support: Even if it seems like a tiny gesture, ask if there is anything you can do to assist. If they need help with daily living duties, social programs, or mental health services, connect them with the proper resources. Make sure their views are heard in the community and the healthcare system by advocating for their needs.

By developing these routines, you may establish a secure and encouraging environment where senior women can express themselves freely and feel heard and understood. Their mental health and overall quality of life may be greatly impacted by the potent instruments of compassion and understanding.

6. Refrain from interjecting or downplaying their worries: Active and focused listening is essential to demonstrating sincere care for an older woman's emotions and ideas. Open-ended inquiries, encouraging cues, summarizing and reflecting, and refraining from interruptions are a few examples.

7. Keep eye contact: Keep eye contact, smile and nod, tuck in your ears, and put away your gadgets. To encourage discourse, choose a peaceful, comfortable area that is free from distractions. Observe their body language and acknowledge their feelings without passing judgment or attempting to make things right.

8. Pay attention to your potential and skills rather than your shortcomings or limits: Emphasize their experiences, resiliency, and wisdom. Express support and encouragement while acknowledging and applauding their accomplishments, no matter how little. This encourages self-worth and confidence.

9. Encourage empathy and good language: Steer clear of judgmental and negative words.

I strongly emphasize on the need of creating a secure and encouraging atmosphere in which older women feel free to express themselves honestly and freely. This entails steering clear of criticism and finger-pointing, encouraging cooperation and teamwork, and recognizing variety and unique experiences.

Concentrating on the physical environment, including making it pleasant, guaranteeing privacy and secrecy, and making it accessible, in order to establish a supportive atmosphere. In order to stop discrimination and harassment, the social environment should be based on trust, inclusion, and well-defined limits.

In addition, the value of speaking inclusively, promoting candid communication, engaging in active listening, and appreciating vulnerability and sincerity are all necessary.I also recommend working with mental health specialists, planning events and activities that are tailored to the interests of women, and giving them access to tools and information on mental health, self-care, and good relationships.

Moreover,it is crucial to protect older women's privacy and confidentiality. They recommend creating safe storage and sharing methods, restricting access to personal data and information to authorized staff only, and seeking express agreement before sharing personal information.

It is important to respect people's physical and emotional limits and to get their consent before touching their possessions or entering restricted areas. Keep proper interpersonal boundaries and be aware of physical touch. Pay attention to their indications and respect their refusal. Be aware of any verbal or nonverbal cues that point to unease or a need for seclusion.

Maintaining confidentiality and privacy standards requires responsibility as well as transparency. They should be honest about who has access to information and how it will be used, give tools for elderly women to view, update, or seek the deletion of their personal information, and clearly explain rules pertaining to data collection, storage, and usage.

In conclusion, by highlighting how crucial it is to provide a space that encourages older women to express themselves honestly and freely. We ought to build a society where every woman may grow psychologically and emotionally by eschewing negativity and placing the blame elsewhere, encouraging cooperation and teamwork, and honoring unique experiences and variety.

Elderly women need to be trusted and respected, and this takes time, steady work, and a dedication to their privacy. It is crucial to think about the possible repercussions of sharing information and balance the advantages against the possibility of invading someone's privacy. Educating senior women about their rights to privacy, offering tools to support them, and encouraging them to speak out if they believe their privacy is being violated will enable them to become stronger advocates for themselves.

To establish trust and preserve older women's dignity, it is essential to respect their physical limits and provide help with tact. Understanding physical limits, honoring personal preferences, observing nonverbal signs, politely giving aid, being aware of personal space, and enabling them to retain independence are important things to keep in mind.

Other recommendations include putting their safety and wellbeing first, understanding cultural variances, speaking succinctly and clearly, and treating everyone with respect and decency. You may make sure that your encounters with older women are considerate of their physical limits, courteous, and supportive by adhering to these principles.

Elderly women's autonomy, well-being, and mental health depend on our accepting their autonomy and capacity for decision-making. Acknowledge their agency and decision-making ability, treat them like mature individuals who can make wise decisions, and provide them the tools and information they need. Refrain from imposing your will on them or making choices on their behalf. Focus on open communication and conversation, embrace them with compassion and understanding, respect their choices—even if they don't align with your own—and provide support without controlling their behavior.

It is essential to provide a secure atmosphere where older women may voice their preferences and concerns without worrying about being judged or rejected. Remind them that you appreciate and cherish their independence. Honor their ability to make decisions, help them reflect on the good and bad outcomes of their choices, and assist them in making wise judgments going forward.

You may disagree with someone's decisions and yet respect their freedom to make them; you don't have to agree with everything they do. Prioritize establishing and preserving relationships of support, resolving disagreements, and creating an atmosphere that is beneficial for everybody.

Recognize that every woman is unique and has various values, objectives, and life experiences in order to embrace variety and uniqueness. It's OK that their decisions will reflect such variances.

You may enable older women to live their lives on their terms, make their own decisions, and actively contribute to society by making these concepts a priority. Advocate for their well-being, adjust your approach and communication style appropriately, and keep up with concerns related to mental health that are unique to older persons. By engaging in these positive behaviors, you may support the development of a culture that values senior women's mental health and wellbeing, promoting dignity and respect and enabling them to enjoy happy, fulfilled lives.

When & How to use resources for mental health of Elderly women

Mood, eating, sleep, and social interaction abnormalities are all indicators of mental health issues in older women. These symptoms may include suicidal thoughts or talk, despair, anxiety, anger, social disengagement, disregard for one's own needs, altered sleep patterns, cognitive abnormalities, delusions, physical changes, and increased alcohol or drug usage.

While not everyone will exhibit every one of these symptoms, it's still vital to pay attention and get treatment from a professional if you have any worries. Supporting older women's mental health requires promoting open conversation and prompt action. Early intervention may have a major impact on the management and course of therapy for mental health issues.

To provide practical support, help older women find a therapist or counselor, help them navigate insurance or financial concerns, frame it as taking care of their overall health, share positive experiences, confront stigma, and encourage older women to seek professional help when they experience ongoing emotional or mental distress. Honor their decisions while highlighting the possible enhancements to their life that expert assistance may provide, such as enhanced coping mechanisms, enhanced relationships, and improved mood.

Be understanding and patient: Change takes time, and there can be obstacles in your path. Be understanding and encouraging to them on their path. You can enable older women to take charge of their mental health and have satisfying lives by normalizing help-seeking, offering helpful assistance, and showing patience and compassion.

It is critical for older women's wellbeing to acknowledge when they need mental health help. You can greatly assist them in navigating their mental health issues and maintaining their mental well-being by being aware of possible indicators and promoting open communication.

Giving older women useful support may make a big difference in their ability to access and use mental health services. Transportation and logistics, emotional and social support, advocacy and guidance, cultural sensitivity, insurance coverage, research possibilities, treatment plans, documentation and forms, and setting up a secure and encouraging environment are examples of practical help.

Particularly for first-time visits, offering to accompany older women to appointments may ease anxiety and provide emotional support. Assist in setting up dependable transportation options, such taxis, trips, or connections to volunteer transport services. Help with appointments and paperwork, including making appointments, filling out papers, and comprehending specifics of insurance coverage.

Senior women may get emotional and social support by establishing a judgment-free, secure environment where they can discuss their experiences and emotions. Making connections with support groups may provide elderly women a feeling of community, shared experiences, and peer support. Assisting them in maintaining their relationships with friends and family may promote happiness and positive social interactions.

Older women who need assistance navigating the healthcare system, comprehending terms and processes, and identifying appropriate caregivers might benefit from advocacy and navigation. Speak out for their needs and, if necessary, put them in touch with financial or legal support. In addition to honoring cultural norms and beliefs, looking for culturally competent therapists, and investigating culturally suitable complementary treatments, cultural issues should be taken into account.

Mental health journeys need patience and tolerance since what works for one woman may not work for another. It is essential to their wellbeing to pay attention to their unique requirements and to provide effective assistance.

Knowing what insurance covers what might assist senior women locate licensed mental health providers that take their insurance or charge reasonable fees. It's crucial to compare treatment options and assist them in selecting the one that most closely matches their demands and financial situation. Assistance is available with appointment scheduling and following up on any testing or referrals.

Helping senior women access mental health services and enhance their well-being requires completing forms together, deciphering medical jargon, and organizing paperwork.

In order to create a safe and supportive environment, one must actively listen without passing judgment, validate their experiences, provide encouragement and support, pay attention to nonverbal signs, respect boundaries, and put them in touch with resources such as support groups or therapy. Recall to honor personal preferences, provide them agency and support within healthcare institutions, and acknowledge and acknowledge their advancements toward mental health.

Chapter 3

The Promoting of Mental
Health by Caregivers

Encouraging Self-Sufficiency and Autonomy

The significance of autonomy and self-sufficiency in caring is examined in this handbook, with a focus on elderly women's mental health. In order to develop independence, resiliency, and a feeling of control over one's life, caregivers are essential. Caregivers make a substantial contribution to the mental health of those they are responsible for by acknowledging and appreciating their strengths. Including elderly women in decision-making processes, assisting them in establishing personal objectives, and giving them chances to express themselves are examples of strategies. In addition to raising self-esteem, this strategy fosters a supportive atmosphere where elderly women feel appreciated and in charge of their life.

This handbook explains how caregivers who support the concepts of self-sufficiency and autonomy may become agents of change for mental health and personal development. Caregivers may be crucial in enabling elderly women to attain long-term mental health and meaningful lives by comprehending and fostering the relationship between self-sufficiency and confidence.

Individuals who take charge of their recovery process are more likely to engage fully in therapy and recovery. Better results and quicker advancement result from this. Enhanced involvement and motivation are essential components of effective mental health treatment. Autonomy and self-sufficiency may increase engagement and motivation through:

1. A feeling of control and ownership: elderly women are more inclined to actively engage in therapy and rehabilitation when they assume responsibility for their own recovery. They also feel more involved in the process. This feeling of ownership strengthens their dedication to their own welfare and sense of duty.

2. Purpose and goal-setting: Being self-sufficient gives elderly women the freedom to decide what their own rehabilitation objectives are and how best to go about achieving them. Their motivation and engagement are fueled by these individualized personal objectives, which are based on their unique needs and desires and provide a feeling of direction and purpose.

3. Enhanced agency and autonomy: Taking charge of decision-making procedures, such as selecting a course of treatment or organizing daily schedules, promotes agency and autonomy. This sense of

empowerment increases drive and promotes involvement in the healing process.

4. Empowerment and self-efficacy: People's confidence in their own talents is bolstered when they acquire new skills and effectively use them to manage their mental health (self-efficacy). Over time, this renewed feeling of empowerment keeps them engaged by igniting their desire to keep learning and developing.

5. Intrinsic rewards and satisfaction: elderly women who practice self-management get intrinsic benefits in the form of enhanced autonomy and well-being as a result of their good experiences.

Collaborative goal-setting, presenting choices and customizing alternatives, concentrating on strengths and developing abilities, encouraging self-advocacy and communication are some strategies used by caregivers to improve motivation and involvement. Through the provision of a supportive atmosphere that encourages self-sufficiency and autonomy, caregivers have the ability to kindle people' drive and involvement, propelling them towards a satisfying life and sustained mental well-being.

In mental health treatment, self-sufficiency and autonomy are critical because they facilitate a smooth transition from caregiver dependency to independent life. This frees up caregivers to concentrate on offering direction and assistance without taking on full control. Self-management abilities, such as effective communication, problem-solving, and emotional control, help elderly women deal with obstacles and get through challenging circumstances on their own, which lessens their need for caregivers for daily assistance and decision-making.

Key advantages of self-sufficiency and autonomy also include increased confidence and self-reliance. Developing self-sufficiency helps elderly women feel more confident about their capacity to take care of their mental health, which lessens their need for outside assistance and direction. Another essential component of autonomy and self-sufficiency is the transfer of accountability and responsibility. Individuals who take charge of their recovery process develop a feeling of maturity and become less dependent on caregivers to make decisions for them by accepting responsibility for their actions.

Healthy boundaries between persons and caregivers guarantee that the right kind of assistance is given without encouraging unhealthy reliance. elderly women are empowered to autonomously manage their self-care while still having access to help when required, thanks to this clear division. The ultimate aims of equipping elderly women with the knowledge and self-assurance to manage their mental health over the long term, encouraging independent living, and lowering the need for ongoing caregiver assistance are long-term sustainability and independence.

By focusing on skill development and knowledge transfer, providing guidance and support, encouraging self-advocacy and empowerment, celebrating autonomy and independence, and giving elderly women the tools and techniques to deal with difficulties and avoid relapse, caregivers can help individuals become less dependent.

Another important result of encouraging self-sufficiency and autonomy in mental health treatment is improved long-term mental health. Self-management skills training and practice provide elderly women the tools and techniques they need to deal with life's obstacles and properly control their symptoms over time, which lessens their dependency on prescription drugs or outside interventions. Long-term stability and greater mental health are also supported by increased resilience and adaptation, which make elderly women more capable of overcoming obstacles in the future and recovering from setbacks.

By emphasizing long-term objectives and sustainability, teaching self-monitoring techniques, encouraging healthy lifestyle choices, putting elderly women in touch with long-term support systems, and fighting for resource access, caregivers may support long-term mental health.

Caregivers can provide elderly women the skills and self-assurance they need to take long-term responsibility for their mental health by encouraging self-sufficiency and autonomy. This will open doors to long-term well-being and a satisfying life. Recall that the path to long-term mental health is an ongoing one, and caregivers may be very helpful in enabling elderly women to travel it with resilience and self-sufficiency.

In order to effectively promote self-sufficiency and autonomy in mental health treatment, a customized strategy that takes into account the particular requirements, skills, and preparedness of each patient is needed. It is critical to comprehend each person's unique requirements since the degree of self-management help required will change based on the severity and complexity of the mental health problem. Self-sufficiency and autonomy may be greatly impacted by a variety of elements, including cognitive and emotional functioning, learning style, cultural and social context, motivation, confidence, capacity for handling responsibilities, and the availability of resources and assistance.

Evaluating someone's motivation, desire for autonomy, and dedication to learning and using self-management techniques are all part of the assessment process. Fostering self-sufficiency requires confidence and self-efficacy, and it is crucial to provide focused assistance to develop these qualities. It's also critical that the person be able to autonomously handle everyday tasks, make wise judgments, and overcome obstacles. Clear limits and a gradual approach may guarantee safe and effective self-management.

Customized treatment plans that address each person's unique requirements, readiness, and learning preferences are created as part of the tailoring process. Flexibility and steady advancement encourage self-sufficiency by introducing more accountability and autonomy in decision-making as the person gains competence and self-assurance. Individuals that participate in collaborative goal setting establish their own self-management objectives, demonstrating their ownership and commitment to their recovery process. The individual's demands are satisfied at every stage of the process toward long-term mental health and self-sufficiency thanks to regular evaluations and modifications.

Caregivers have the ability to customize their assistance and encourage self-reliance in a manner that enables elderly women to successfully manage their mental health and enjoy satisfying lives. In order to promote self-sufficiency and autonomy in mental health treatment, it is imperative that reliance be addressed. Determining the primary source of reliance helps in customizing efficient therapies. Overdependence may hinder development, sap motivation, and make it more difficult to manage mental health.

Open communication and teamwork, concentrating on strengths and capabilities, gradually reducing support, skill-building and knowledge transfer, positive reinforcement and encouragement, setting clear boundaries and expectations, and encouraging access to additional resources are some strategies for addressing dependency. In order to address dependence, one must provide the person the tools they need to take long-term responsibility for their mental health rather than abandoning them.

Throughout the process, be understanding and patient while providing constant encouragement and support. Working together with the patient and other medical providers to develop a customized strategy that meets their unique requirements and encourages steady development toward self-reliance is essential. Caregivers may help elderly women take control of their mental health and have satisfying lives by addressing reliance in a healthy way and teaching self-management skills.

Pursuing self-sufficiency requires ensuring one's health and safety. There should be support networks and well-defined boundaries. In order to promote self-sufficiency and autonomy in mental health care, a collaborative partnership where the patient is empowered to take charge of their own journey and the caregiver acts as a supportive guide and navigator is needed, rather than downplaying the importance of caregivers. Fostering the confidence and abilities necessary for self-management allows caregivers to provide persons the resources they need to live happy, independent lives.

Addressing Mental Health Issues in Caregivers

Caregivers face numerous challenges in their role, including stress, burnout, and emotional exhaustion. These challenges can significantly impact the well-being of both the caregiver and the person they care for. Chronic stress can lead to fatigue, headaches, digestive issues, anxiety, and sleep problems, while emotional exhaustion can result from witnessing a loved one's struggles and managing their own emotions. This can lead to cynicism, detachment, and difficulty finding meaning in their role.

Stress and burnout can also strain relationships with the person being cared for and other family members, as well as personal relationships, work life, and overall quality of life. To combat stress and burnout, caregivers should prioritize self-care by committing time to activities that nourish their physical and mental well-being, such as exercise, meditation, spending time in nature, hobbies, socializing with friends, or getting enough sleep.
Seek professional help from therapists or counselors experienced in caregiver stress and burnout to equip them with coping mechanisms, stress management techniques, and emotional

support. Practice mindfulness and relaxation techniques to manage stress and promote emotional resilience. Set boundaries and say no to additional demands and delegate tasks whenever possible to protect time and energy. Build a support network by connecting with other caregivers online or in person to share experiences, find understanding, and access resources.

Utilize community resources like respite care, adult day care programs, or home help services to provide temporary relief and allow caregivers to recharge. Communicate openly with your loved one and other family members about your needs and challenges to help everyone understand the situation and find solutions together.

Secondary trauma is another significant concern for caregivers, as witnessing and supporting someone experiencing mental health challenges can take a toll on their own mental well-being. Understanding secondary trauma involves empathizing with and supporting their loved ones, leading to an involuntary emotional response known as emotional contagion. Over time, repeated exposure to trauma can lead to symptoms similar to post-traumatic stress disorder (PTSD) in caregivers.

Protecting yourself from secondary trauma involves maintaining awareness and education about its potential, setting boundaries and limiting exposure, practicing self-care and emotional hygiene, seeking professional help from therapists or counselors, building a support network, and acknowledging that secondary trauma is a real and valid experience. Taking care of oneself is essential for protecting one's mental health and effectively supporting their loved one.

Caregivers often prioritize their loved ones' needs over their own, **neglecting their physical and mental health**. This neglect can lead to physical decline, emotional burnout, increased stress and anxiety, reduced immunity, and increased vulnerability. To prioritize self-care as a caregiver, schedule self-care activities into your routine, block time for exercise, relaxation, hobbies, or social connection, and start small and build gradually. Pay attention to your body and prioritize rest, relaxation, or activities that help you de-stress when feeling fatigued, stressed, or overwhelmed. Communicate and delegate: Don't be afraid to ask for help from family, friends, or community resources about sharing caregiving responsibilities or providing respite care. Focus on progress, not perfection, and forgive yourself for setbacks.

Remember that self-care is not a luxury; it's a necessity. By taking care of yourself, you'll be better equipped to care for your loved one and maintain your own physical and mental well-being.

Social isolation is another challenge for caregivers. The intense demands of caregiving can often lead to a gradual separation from social circles, leaving caregivers feeling alone and disconnected. The grip of social isolation includes limited time and energy, fear of burdening others, misunderstood experiences, and loss of identity beyond caregiving. Strategies for breaking through social isolation include starting small and seeking micro-connections, communicating openly about your needs, seeking out caregiver-specific communities, reconnecting with personal interests, and using technology to stay connected.

Promoting caregiver mental health involves seeking professional help from therapists or counselors experienced in supporting caregivers. They can equip you with coping mechanisms, stress management techniques, and emotional support. Prioritize self-care by making time for activities you enjoy, even if it's just for a short while each day. Exercise, meditation, spending time in nature, and healthy hobbies can contribute to well-being.

Build a support network by connecting with other caregivers online or in person to share experiences, find understanding, and learn from each other. Support groups provide a safe space and a sense of community. Set boundaries between your role as caregiver and your personal life by saying no when needed and delegating tasks whenever possible. Communicate openly: Talk to your loved one about your own needs and feelings. Open communication can help both of you cope with the challenges of the situation.

In conclusion, prioritizing self-care as a caregiver is essential for maintaining overall well-being and preventing loneliness. By scheduling self-care activities into your routine, starting small and building consistency, listening to your body, communicating openly, and utilizing technology to stay connected, caregivers can break through social isolation and lead more fulfilling lives.

"As you close this guide, take a moment to reflect on your journey through its pages." Recognize the obstacles you've overcome, enjoy your accomplishments, and look forward to the opportunities that await you. Remember that mental health is a journey, not a destination. Continue to study, try new things, and figure out what feeds your mind, body, and soul. May the year 2024 be one of increasing self-awareness and unshakable self-compassion."